MY ROAD
TO
FERTILITY

OLUWATOSIN ADEBANJO-ORE

Copyright © 2022
OLUWATOSIN ADEBANJO-ORE

Designed by:
Print Doctor Africa Ltd
Plot 10 Block A Area 4 OPIC Estate,
Agbara
www.printdoctorafrica.com

DEDICATION

This book is dedicated to God Almighty, the Author and Finisher of my faith, my loving husband, Omolade, my son, Oluwabamise, (God did it for me), all the women in waiting and my late dad, Prince Adedoyin Stephen Adebanjo who unfortunately passed on four months before the birth of my baby.

ACKNOWLEDGEMENT

My sincere gratitude goes to the rest of my cheerleading team, my mum, siblings, parent in-laws, in-laws, cousins, aunties, uncles and friends who were with me throughout the journey. Lastly, to the five beautiful women who agreed to share their stories through this book.

TABLE OF CONTENTS

"I am learning to trust the journey even when I do not understand it."

Mila Bron

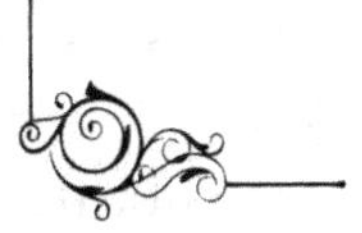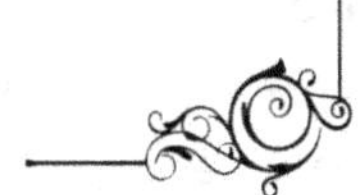

MY STORY

Infertility is nothing to be ashamed of. Many women waiting to conceive tend to shy away from living their lives thereby putting it on hold. Societal pressure, family interference, and not knowing how to deal with comments publicly contribute to women hiding themselves and wallowing in pity. This is a big mistake and a misconception that affects women trying to conceive. You don't control your body or yourself. I think it is wrong that nobody wants to talk about this topic.

The motivation behind this book is my promise to God to tell my story and share my testimony to encourage any woman going through fertility issues. I am sharing my story because I have been there, and I know how those currently going through infertility may feel. Women don't have to endure or struggle with infertility silently.

There is this unspoken norm to avoid sharing stories or remain quiet when it comes to infertility especially in the society we live in as people feel it creates discomfort as a topic.

My journal was a place of solace and comfort, which I frequently engaged even before I got pregnant. Every appointment, schedule, date, event, occasion including little details were carefully documented as I had the conviction that I was going to go back to my journal and tell my story. This allowed me to open up more about the topic, as I have always loved writing. A few of my friends would ask me "how far" or "se o ti wole" (has it entered) and my response then was that we were still trying, especially if I felt the question or concern was genuine. In most cultures in Nigeria, once you have been married for a couple of months without getting pregnant, people would start to wonder what is wrong with you. You attend weddings or outings and everyone has an opinion about what you should be doing to get pregnant. Don't get me wrong, people that genuinely care will pray for you or with you or even ask you what is wrong. It is tough for women trying to conceive especially when there is a lot of societal pressure and family interference. There is a lot of pressure already in trying to get pregnant, I mean the consultations, medication, prayers, advice, work, and life in general is enough but at the same time, you get advice to be calm and not think about it as it will occur naturally.

I hope sharing my story will encourage others and allow people to talk openly about infertility, support, and simply be there for each other.

An important tool for this journey is the beautiful word called 'faith'. One of our favourite phrases that kept us motivated is by Adel Bestavros 'Patience with God is faith, patience with self is hope, and patience with others is love'. Having faith in God is being patient with God's plan and timing. We held on to this as we prayed daily. My husband and I always had faith in God. We had faith that we were going to carry our children but having faith in God does not stop you from doing your research. James 2:14-18 says:

What good is it, my brothers and sisters, if someone claims to have faith but has no deeds? Can such faith save them? 15 Suppose a brother or a sister is without clothes and daily food. 16 If one of you says to them, "Go in peace; keep warm and well fed," but does nothing about their physical needs, what good is it? 17 In the same way, faith by itself, if it is not accompanied by action, is dead. 18 But someone will say, "You have faith; I have deeds. "Show me your faith without deeds, and I will show you my faith by my deeds.

Having God beside us all through the journey was a great reassurance, and having a team of specialists also gave direction and reignited our hope as faith and work will give results.

We got engaged in December 2013 and got married a year after in December 2014.

Our wedding was glamorous, and we had about 1500 guests in attendance. I remember it being a happy day with a lot of dancing and prayers. It was like a dream come true, and like the average woman, I calculated that I was going to conceive before the end of the following year (2015). It reminds me of the saying, "Man proposes God disposes". You cannot claim supremacy over God; whatever comes out as a result of man's intelligent pursuit cannot be claimed as his own doing without God's intervention.

After the wedding and whole honeymoon phase, I had to go back to Dubai to continue teaching without my husband as we were still thinking of the best plan going forward. He was based in Nigeria at the time. Going back to Dubai after our wedding was tough on both of us as we had to plan when to visit each other.

During the first two years of our marriage, we just continued being best friends and bonding. The time difference was 5 hours, so we were always on Skype (this was before Dubai banned Skype). We would talk, and video call on Skype for hours. We didn't think there were any issues regarding conceiving. Being a teacher made it easier as there was time off work every 2 to 3 months. I travelled frequently to Nigeria and would typically go to Lagos like four times a year to see my hubby. On the other hand, he would come to Dubai during shorter holidays, and sometimes, we would travel to the US or a resort in another emirate in the United Arab Emirates. Summer time meant spending two months with him, two weeks for spring, and three weeks for the winter holiday, so I was not particularly worried, thinking the lack of us not living together caused the delay. Prior to this, I never calculated my ovulation period because I didn't even know how to. My sister introduced me to an app to start tracking my ovulation. I downloaded the app but never really bothered to use it.

Looking back now, God's time is never late because the period we waited made us closer to each other. There was no parental pressure from both sides as we just continued living in the moment and getting to know ourselves even more. There were a couple of people who would tease us about when we will have children, but we would just laugh about it. In addition, anytime I went to Nigeria and attended weddings or functions, I would get a couple of people (especially older people) praying for us while some would stare openly at my tummy.

August 2016

My husband finally moved to Dubai, and we started trying to track my ovulation using the ovulation app I had downloaded. The months in between had seen us living purely apart and we saw for about 3 weeks during the Easter holidays which we spent in the States with family.

Funny tip- *I had read online somewhere that you should lay on your back with legs up high so the swimmers can go in deeper and not slide back out. LOL. Things we do when looking for pikin. Well, I did it and my husband looked at me strangely when I refused to get up and used my hands to hold my legs up high, Please don't think in picture. I know I did and I am not the first woman to be caught in that position, hahaha.*

December 2016

I felt excruciating pain in my tummy and could barely stand up straight. My assumption was the regular period pain; when it didn't subdue, I visited a gynaecologist. After a series of questions and examinations, she suspected fibroids. She suggested I do some scans, which confirmed her suspicions. Alas! I had a couple of fibroids.

Some days later, my gynaecologist told me about the effect of this on me trying to get pregnant. There was a large one resting on my uterus, and she advised me to remove it to avoid it blocking my chances of having children due to its location. She told many positive stories about numerous women who removed fibroids and still got pregnant within a year. Instead of fear, I remember getting excited, thinking that pregnancy would be next once the fibroids were removed. She explained the process of fibroid removal and how long it takes to recuperate. As a teacher with summer holiday, I was already calculating the best time to do the surgery. July was the best option as there was a long break giving me adequate time to heal and recover.

July 2017

Six months have gone by since the diagnosis. Within the twinkle of an eye, the much awaited time has come. I am about to go under the knife for the first time. The surgery I was to undergo is called a laparoscopic myomectomy. A couple of small incisions is made in or near your navel. Then a laparoscope is inserted. A laparoscope is a narrow tube fitted with a camera into your abdomen where the fibroids are then cut and removed. I was told to fast at least 12 hours before.

Mixed emotions of fear, anxiety and excitement for the prospects of conception filled my mind. On that fateful morning, we drove to the hospital with our bags packed for the weekend as if we were headed to a fancy resort. One funny detail was how I called my husband, held his hands, and told him all my bank card's passwords. He looked at me puzzled and asked why, then I said the silliest thing ever. "In case I don't make it out" he laughed, kissed me on the forehead, reassured me, and said, "Don't be silly, see you in a few hours" I was taken in to get prepped, all jewelleries and personal belongings were taken off and handed to my husband. As I was wheeled in, a cloud of emotions rushed over me. Was I overthinking? Or was it as serious? Regardless, I had never had a surgery, so I wasn't sure how I felt.

Laying on my back and looking up in the theatre, all I saw were white lights everywhere around me. The doctor came to my side after I had gotten anaesthetic. She reassured me that everything would be fine and asked me to count to 10. 1,2,3,4…… beep beep beep were the sounds I heard hours after as I opened my eyes. I knew where I was immediately and remembered I just had a surgery. I was in a lot of pain and couldn't talk.

While being wheeled out, my husband approached earnestly, and I thought I was talking, but the words never came out. After a while, I softly mumbled "I'm I'm I'm in pains, and a tear dropped from his eyes as he leaned over to kiss my forehead. My husband was so supportive during my recovery and literally did everything for me from cooking to cleaning and running errands too. My parents and siblings called to speak to me immediately as they were all anxious and concerned. My mum wanted to fly down as she was in the US at the time but we assured her we were fine. Now, when you remove fibroids, the recovery time is about 6 to 8 weeks, and you are advised not to have sex during this period. Slowly and gradually I got better, healing was taking place in my mind and body. It's the middle of summer and there was so much to do but the doctor said no sex and no stressful activity. One of my friends was getting married that summer and it was one of the events to look forward to. We attended looking fly but due to my gradual recovery, I was unable to wear heels. The wedding was colourful and eventful as there was a lot of eat, drink and the presence of good company. At some point, I felt some pain and had to sit down as I had been standing and dancing for too long. There was an awkward moment where someone tried to hand me a baby to carry for a few minutes while she sorted some things out. I didn't tell her I had a surgery and was not ready to start explaining. Luckily, my sister in-law was right beside me and immediately rose to help with the baby. According to my doctor's advice, I was told not to carry anything above a certain weight or mass including a baby.

Tip- *We may find ourselves in an awkward situation where we can't explain or don't feel like explaining. It is okay to do you. People that like you may not need an explanation and people that don't like you may not believe you.*

We had a blissful but quiet summer. We were mostly Netflix and chilling and I had to be careful with movie selection so as not to arouse my hungry roommate.

2018

We continued trying for a baby. Everything was normal, but I was still not pregnant though we had been trying since I recovered from the surgery. A lot of our friends didn't think we were trying for a baby, probably because we stayed positive and not gloomy.

Our worries remained in our hearts and not in our disposition. Thank God for a God-fearing husband, and maybe I should say both our faith was so strong that we knew once God is ready to give us children, He will do it at the right time. All this time, I joined the children's church and never allowed myself to wallow in pity. I would celebrate and dance forward during baby dedication thanksgiving and tap into people's blessings. Having our own child was our main prayer point. After a while, we just started thanking God because we believed our prayer had been answered and what we were waiting for was just the 'when'. . I actually loved being around children. I was a teacher by profession while also volunteering in the church.

In February, my sister moved to Canada and persuaded us to apply for permanent residency. To be honest, we were quite comfortable in Dubai and didn't see the need to move to Canada. One thing she said that resonated with us and made us change our minds was the fact that Ontario had free IVF for couples amongst other juicy prospects. A few months into 2018, we decided to apply for permanent residency in Canada. On January 4, 2019, our application was approved, and we became permanent residents of Canada. We had done our research extensively and decided to move to Toronto.

March 2019

A new phase begins. We moved to Toronto in our 5th year of marriage. After researching and visiting a few clinics, we finally registered with a family doctor close to our home. Our first consultation with our doctor was about a month after. We told him we had been trying for a baby for a couple of years. He asked us a couple of questions before referring us to a fertility doctor, but alas! The next appointment the fertility doctor had was December 2019, which was 5 months after. He assured us that the fertility doctor was really good and it would be worth the wait.

December 2019

A day we will never forget. We met the fertility doctor and discussed with him for about an hour. God bless him. He made us feel at ease and kept telling me I was still quite young. I smiled every time he said that because 36 is not young at all and simply because everything I had read online had to do with risks from 35 years of age, or maybe it was just part of his process of making patients feel at ease but trust me it worked.

He carefully explained the process and tests we had to do (which was a lot). He backed most of his work/process with statistics. I was comfortable with this doctor because he was quite reassuring and confident (also because I always feel comfortable with doctors who are more advanced in age). He went on to tell us IVF was usually the last resort for him as it is invasive. We spoke for about an hour and we asked a ton of questions. He patiently answered all our questions and assured us that I will get pregnant.

The treatment started and I was subjected to give blood samples which was used to run about 20 tests. They tested my husband's semen to check for low sperm count, amongst other things. He told us to come back in a month to discuss the results of the blood work.

A couple of weeks later, we went back to see the doctor. The doctor prescribed DHEA, folic acid, COQ0, and PQQ. He asked that I continue to use these drugs indefinitely. The cost of these medications was about 300 dollars monthly. I was taking about 10 tablets in total daily.

Fun fact: *I am one of those people who have no issues with pills or tablets. Funnily enough, I could take a bunch of tablets together with little or no water. At this point, taking about ten pills a day for months was exhausting but I had to keep going as I kept my eyes on the goal.*

February 2020

I did an endometrial biopsy at the clinic. This is a medical procedure in which a small piece of tissue from the lining of the uterus is removed for examination under a microscope. The tissue removed is viewed to look for abnormal cells. I was asked to take ibuprofen 30 minutes before the procedure. It was quite painful and uncomfortable. A suction catheter was inserted through my cervix into the uterine cavity for this. After the procedure, I had mild cramping and spotting.

After this procedure, I was told to take Letrozole for five days. The doctor requested a blood test and ultrasound, and fortunately, my follicle count was good. The next step involved an injection called HCG to ovulate. This is administered when you produce healthy eggs. The doctor told us when to have sex and told me to buy a pregnancy kit, and with fingers crossed, this may work. The two-week wait was the longest 2 weeks ever. Unfortunately, I tested negative afterwards. My heart was broken as I was sure this was it. We talked about it, prayed, and dusted ourselves up for the next round.

I remember on our first meeting; the doctor showed us a road map. It was the sequence to his treatment. He detailed all the procedures and steps he would take and the expected outcome per stage. If per chance, the outcome was negative, we would proceed to the next step, which was usually more intensive and delicate. The last step was usually IVF which he would perform if all previous steps failed.

April 2020

At the height of the Covid-19 outbreak, fertility clinics closed indefinitely, so all appointments were cancelled until further notice. To manage this disappointment and not have a cluster of negative thoughts and lethargy, I downloaded an exercise app and started daily exercise. I needed all the strength I could muster at this stage, and I found it in listening to soul-nourishing gospel music. Thankfully, my husband had a lovely playlist, and I fell in love with a particular song that spoke to me daily. The best part of music for me is always content. As well as I appreciate rhythm; the content is what leaves the impact (Hillsong 'I Surrender' and 'Seasons') were my songs for the period. The song 'Seasons' is worthy of being shared because it inspired hope and helped rebuild my faith when doubt, anxiety or fear crept in.

Like the frost on a rose
Winter comes for us all
Oh how nature acquaints us
With the nature of patience
Like a seed in the snow
I've been buried to grow
For Your promise is loyal
From seed to sequoia
I know
Though the winter is long even richer
The harvest it brings
Though my waiting prolongs even greater
Your promise for me like a seed
I believe that my season will come
Lord I think of Your love
Like the low winter sun
And as I gaze I am blinded
In the light of Your brightness
And like a fire to the snow
I'm renewed in Your warmth
Melt the ice of this wild soul

'Til the barren is beautiful
And I know
Though the winter is long even richer
The harvest it brings
Though my waiting prolongs even greater
Your promise for me like a seed
I believe that my season will come
I can see the promise
I can see the future
you're the God of seasons
And I'm just in the winter
If all I know of harvest
Is that it's worth my patience
Then if You're not done working
God I'm not done waiting
You can see my promise
Even in the winter
'Cause You're the God of greatness
Even in a manger
For all I know of seasons
Is that You take Your time
You could have saved us in a second
Instead You sent a child, oh
Though the winter is long even richer
The harvest it brings
Though my waiting prolongs even greater
Your promise for me like a seed
I believe that my season will come
And when I finally see my tree
Still I believe there's a season to come
Like a seed You were sown

For the sake of us all
From Bethlehem's soil
Grew Calvary's sequoia
Source: LyricFind
Songwriters: Ben Tan / Benjamin William Hastings /
Chris Davenport

June 2020

Two months after, I remember getting a call from my mum in America telling me she heard fertility clinics in Ontario have reopened. How did my mum even know this all the way from the US? This information was thrilling to hear. She advised calling my doctor to confirm. Without wasting time, the clinic was called, and an appointment was booked for the end of June.

My greatest discomfort every time I visited the clinic was having my blood sample taken. Looking for my vein to get blood drawn has always been an issue. Unfortunately for me, when the fertility clinic reopened, there was a new phlebotomist. She always had to call the head nurse as she never could locate my vein, so I ended up spending extra time there. During this period, I was getting my blood drawn weekly.

The next stage of my treatment started on June 29th, 2020. The doctor ordered a blood test and ultrasound to be done. Letrozole was prescribed for me again. This time, my doctor told me to take it for three days. Five on day one; three on day two, and two on day three.

One thing about Letrozole is that it has to be taken at the exact time each day. For instance, 3pm is 3pm and not 3.01pm. This little fact got me teased by my husband as he says I am too formal and by the books. My experience trying to conceive also added to my knowledge of sieving what you read on Google.

Going online, for example, and reading that the dosage for Letrozole was one every day for 5 days. I told my doctor, but he said it was okay to take it in three days as it would hasten the process.

Tip- *Online doctors and Google prescriptions are not proper consultations. Please always talk to a proper doctor or filter what you read online as you may read meaning to things that are not an issue.*

July 3rd, 2020

I had a sonohysterogram done today. This is a procedure where the doctor takes a look at the inside of your uterus. It helps to diagnose many problems that lead to infertility. It uses sound waves to produce pictures of the inside to a woman's uterus. I was told to take Advil about 30 minutes before and to empty my bladder too. They found a 7cm fibroid and some other small ones, but unlike the fibroid I had some years ago, this was nowhere close to my uterus. The doctor advised my hubby and me to have sex on Sunday and Monday, then booked a follow-up appointment on Tuesday.

July 7, 2020

I had an ultrasound, and they gave me an HCG injection. This injection stimulates the release of eggs during ovulation. HCG stimulates the ovaries and helps a woman's eggs to mature and be released into the woman's ovarian tubes and then into the uterus.
So, I was told to have sex a day and 2 days after my HCG injection. This HCG injection I took clashes with my ovulation date. Hmmmmm….This one na twins loading ooo.

July 16, 2020.

I felt very bloated, and it seemed as if I was peeing a lot. Fingers crossed. Went for another appointment. Blood test was done, and I was asked to come back in a week for a pregnancy test. I was curious and did a pregnancy test at home on Monday but it was negative. I felt disappointed but as my brothers say "we move".

Thursday, July 23, 2020

On my way to the clinic for a test, I decided to read messages from a female group I belong to, and they are talking about fertility. Reading so many stories made me feel a certain peace that God will do it for us, and we will share our testimony.

My appointments were now weekly as opposed to monthly. I opted for early morning (6.45 am appointments, so I could still go to work from there. I had support from colleagues who stood in for me in my absence. My teammates were always willing to stay for a couple of minutes in my classroom if running late. My supervisor would always tell me that they usually have at least two staff get pregnant yearly. Coincidentally, the same year I started at the job, there were already 3 women on maternity leave, so I tapped into that too.

I was determined and prayed to God not to do this for more than a month as it was stressful. On appointment days, I would wake up super early to make my trip down to the clinic before 6.45am, then get a large syringe in my veins to draw blood, after then, an ultrasound before meeting with the doctor weekly. This was the cycle every appointment day. On this particular day, while heading to my doctor, someone close to me said something insensitive. The person asked when I would get pregnant. My response to her was "Do you even know if and why I am not pregnant"? You see people often say insensitive things, maybe not intentionally but saying certain things especially not knowing what an individual may be going through is not nice. Being a frequent visitor of a specialist doctor is like a bad car and a mechanics' relationship, having blood drawn from my tiny and almost invisible veins, ingesting tons of pills and medication of various sizes, shapes and colours, waking up early for those appointments, balancing this with work and other life issues is tough enough without an insensitive jest or remarks about my situation.

Monday, July 27, 2020

Follow up appointment with an ultrasound and blood test done. Letrozole was prescribed for me to take again for three days. I remember praying and playing the song 'Seasons' by Hill song in the car repeatedly. My birthday was two days before (July 25). It is good to profess what you want with your mouth to God and talking to God sure makes a difference. I prophesized that I wanted to have my own child by my next birthday. My family organized a zoom birthday party for me and most of the prayers had to do with us conceiving before the year runs out. Whenever anyone prays for me, you would hear a resounding amen from me, you just never know when there is a spirit nearby.

August 6, 2020.

I went to the fertility clinic to take an HCG injection. Couple of days after taking this injection my legs hurt like crazy, felt bloated and had serious cramps. My hubby give me massages to make it better. Trust me the right partner matters in this journey.

With all this, I was still taking my daily medication of DHEA, PQQ, COQ10 and folic acid.

August 13, 2020

On this day, I was told my progesterone level is good. Yipeee!! The little things that excite one in this journey. Finally!! Maybe this is going to be it.

August 20, 2020

The weird thing about this journey is you have to go in to the clinic whenever you are on your period too. An ultrasound and blood test is usually performed. Being an optimistic and positive person, I felt overwhelmed with everything for the first time ever, woke up at 3am and felt exhausted. Mehn! The devil is a liar, after waiting for this long, this distraction and down feeling is not for me at all. My husband woke up and we prayed together. That particular day was hard as I contemplated pausing the treatment temporarily. God reminded me of my prayer two days after my birthday to wait till exactly a month after which was August 27. It was just August 20, so I still had 7 days technically. I moved my appointment to August 25.

My road to fertility made me realize the importance of asking questions. Reading has always been my favourite thing to do so researching came to me easily. Before going to the clinic weekly I would have read so many things online (filtered of course) because if you are not careful, you would end up reading things that may get you apprehensive. Reading stuff during the week made me write so many questions down and asking so many questions at every appointment gave me a lot of clarity on all procedure.

Another important thing is to continue your life the same way and not let negativity get to you. The society we live in is a cruel one. You will hear all sorts! People gossiping, backbiting. Spreading rumours etc. To think about it, one of the funniest things I heard then was that I couldn't have a child as this was even news to me. There was a day, someone called me in church and just prayed with me; now knowing this person was genuine touched me and opening up wasn't so hard. She was surprised and told me and I quote "God bless you Tosin, please continue to radiate and light up everywhere you go with your beautiful smile, you are blessed and you don't know it" she also said she never knew we were trying for a baby based on our attitude and how involved we were. Ladies trying to conceive, please don't stop living your life. This brings me to an incident where someone told me not to post on social media because people will be wondering why I am gallivanting instead of thinking of how to have a baby. This surprised me and my next question was "how do people that want babies behave? Of course, she immediately got defensive and said she was just telling me what someone said about me. When people are comfortable speaking to your friends about you, then there is a problem. Note that you are not living your life for people as humans are quick to judge without looking inward. Another one of my acquaintances told me she was always zooming all my pictures on social media to check if I was pregnant. I just laughed and told her to continue zooming because one day, she will actually zoom and see a bump.

There was an incident where someone I just met asked me how my kids were. Being a teacher, I refer to my students as my kids so in casual conversation, my default response is they are fine especially when I am talking to someone I don't have a relationship with. Then she probed further but since it was our first time meeting, I wasn't too comfortable discussing details so we kept chatting until she pushed the button. During the course of our conversation, I had mentioned to her that I don't have children and I had been married for five years. She dropped the ball when she asked me, "what are you doing about it? The question felt rude, crude, too direct and presumptuous. I did not like it especially as I didn't know her. At this point, I got tired of smiling and felt there was no point in engaging her any further as it seemed she was simply probing and not casually engaging in a friendly conversation.

On my road to fertility, the realization that people don't know what to actually say to family or friends waiting to conceive dawned on me. Maybe once upon a time, I was guilty of the same. Going through infertility was an eye opener for me as I discovered it's a conversation that exists but only those affected engage in it. Don't get me wrong, it is okay to talk to friends or family about it only and I repeat, only if it is coming from a good place.

There were people that were actually concerned but didn't know how to talk about it with me but will say a prayer or ask indirectly, this also touched me and I would usually assure whoever we are on it.

Many a times, there are strange and somewhat embarrassing situations and conversations where people say weird things or insensitive things that may trigger emotions of someone going through infertility, however when I sensed genuine care or concern, it was always easy to respond and it was not awkward. There was an occasion where I met the mother of a friend for the first time. The sweet old lady assumed I had a child and extended regards to my baby. So when I responded that I didn't have a child yet, she looked at me and said,' I understand. Then she held my hands and prayed with me. After that she shared her story and apparently, she also waited for 10 years before conception. Frankly, I felt a connection with her as she was warm and genuine. No tears, no pity party, no sad faces but good vibes, good energy and my faith was revived from that one encounter with her.

August 25, 2020

Another appointment and I was happy because my uterine lining had thickened and my follicles had reached the required size and deemed ready for egg collection. At this point, my doctor told me a HCG trigger shot (which induces ovulation about 36 hours after the injection) will be given and will schedule my IUI. Letrozole was prescribed for 3 days after which I was told to come back on August 31.

August 31, 2020

I had a follow up visit at the clinic today and was given a herculean task. After pleasantries and friendly chats, the nurse looked at me and told me something I wasn't sure I heard right. She said, "this is a trigger injection which you must use on yourself tonight. Hold up! Can you repeat that? LOL. My Ijebu self translated it in my native language 'Yoruba' (kin gun ara mi ni abere) translation " I should inject myself? How is that even going to work? I hate needles and pain, yet I am to inflict it on myself and right in my belly. Is there no alternative? To paint a vivid picture of how it went down, this was the conversation between myself and the nurse:

Tosin: I can't do it Lucy, you know how much I hate needles, what other option is available.

Nurse: (Laughing) Tosinnnnn, you have to try or tell your hubby.

Tosin: Hubby has never given an injection before and doesn't know how to.

Nurse: Do you want us to try this process next month?

Tosin: Looking at her with side eye, Lucy, don't try me o (we were really cool by the way and we always cracked jokes with each other all the time)

Nurse: Do you want to do a zoom call if it will make you feel better?

Tosin: Okay, I will set one up.

Fortunately, I didn't have to do that as your girl braved up and got injected in the belly later on that night by my husband.

The trigger shot ensures mature eggs are released in 36-40 hours. Based on this, I was told to come back two days after for an IUI. I asked about the success rate based on my age and also as this is the first time. Guess what? This procedure guarantees only a 10 percent chance of getting pregnant at the first try due to my age. I smiled and initially doubted but remembered God's word in Proverbs 3.5

Trust in the Lord with all your heart

The next two days got me reading and researching as much possible. The thirst to know everything about IUI was so intense, my husband on the other hand was so sure I would get pregnant. To take my mind off it, he booked a getaway for us a few days after the IUI. We were advised to abstain from sex before IUI.

September 2, 2020

I woke up refreshed, thankful but at the same time nervous. Knowing what to expect every step of the way but still anxious.

A typical IUI cycle begins at the start of your period and ends when you take a blood pregnancy test, about two weeks after your IUI.

When we got there, my husband's sample sperm was collected and washed. The sperm wash helps to eliminate weak sperm, bacteria etc. It concentrates the motile sperm to ensure a large number gets to the uterus. It also separates the sperm cells from the seminal fluid. After the sperm was collected and during the washing, we went to a mall close by to just walk around, window shop and just talk as we were told to come back in an hour for the procedure.

After an hour, we went back to the clinic. The nurse took us into a room and told me to lay down. The process was explained to us in detail and then my doctor inserted a speculum into me and thread a thin, flexible catheter through my cervix to deposit my husband's sperm into my uterus.

The entire process took about 5 minutes. My doctor put me at ease and cracked me up when she said these sperm are so clean, now let's see which of these twenty five million swimmers would get to the Promised Land first. After the procedure, she advised I lay down for about 10 minutes to prevent me from feeling lightheaded or dizzy. What came to my mind instead was "hmmm, maybe she wants me to lie down so the sperm could go in properly because I read somewhere that even after having sex sometimes, you should raise your legs up. Things we see online.

2 week wait-The Niagara Falls escape

Some days after the IUI procedure, the doctor summoned me to do a pregnancy test. This was done and thus began my anxiety journey. To get my mind off it, we booked a getaway for a couple of days. I was tempted to do a self-test but decided against it. The pressure of the procedure and anxiety of the result coming almost sipped out the joy and excitement of Niagara Falls. We got a suite with a Jacuzzi overlooking the falls from a very close distance. Everything seemed perfect and my husband was loving the ambience but I was so distracted. In the midst of any happy times, I would daydream and get lost in my reverie. Uncertainty, anxiety, and thoughts of the next step if this failed could not stop bullying me. Snap out of it Tosin- I would say to myself but I was right back after some moments.

After a lovely breakfast, we walked to the falls and started our day. We saw the water, went down the tunnels, explored the city, took tours, and just enjoyed the sights and sounds.

For some reason, I was extra careful. That evening, the hubby took me out for a lovely steak dinner. I had on a beautiful short dress and white sneakers. After our meal, we decided to walk to the amusement park area. It was so beautiful and had a Las Vegas look and feel. Lights, rides, wax museums, music and yes ice cream. From a distance my husband spotted a bridge with lights and got excited. It was a go-kart track, we walked down and he so eagerly wanted to get on the ride but I was in a vibe-killer mood as I refused. I begged him to consider as I wore a short dress and told him I would like to go back to the hotel to change and then we could come back to that side of town,

Back at the room, we opened a bottle of champagne to celebrate, turned on some soft music and got into the Jacuzzi. It was barely a few minutes and I was done. I wanted out. For some strange reasons, I felt dizzy. My husband looked at me in disbelief, I had refused to drink. I refused the go-kart and next thing I said was sleep time. He was upset as I was truly living the vibe killer mantra.

For most women, this "two-week wait" is the hardest part of the IUI cycle. It can be tempting to read into every symptom you experience. Do your sore breasts mean you're about to get your period? Or does it mean that you're pregnant? Only the blood test will offer official confirmation.

Sept 15, 2020

We got back from our holiday and got a call from the clinic. I put the call on speaker as I didn't know what to expect. It was from the head nurse who was so excited she had to make the call herself. She broke the best news of all time to us. We were numb and shocked. We didn't know what to do or how to react. We just got on our knees and started thanking God.

This was it, I had suddenly become a pregnant woman. Is this it? Seven years of constant compounding sex, 7 years of anxiety, uncertainty, research, injections, surgery, hospitals, specialists and medication. Is this the end of my infertility? I was wowed yet I had questions. It felt so easy and I made a deep sigh of relief after the call. Tears did not flow like I thought they would as I did not shed a single tear after hearing the news.

God did it. As I sank into the couch with my husband beside me, we kept looking into each other's eyes but could not find the words to express how we felt. The clinic just confirmed I was 5 weeks pregnant but an air of doubt passed through our minds as we could not fathom how God did it when we least expected it as we thought it will be more complex especially as the specialist had informed us the probability of success was just ten percent. The song that came to mind and we kept singing was 'Were lo bami se'' (He did it with ease).

"We do not 'get over' a death.

We learn to carry the grief and integrate the loss in our lives. In our hearts, we carry those who have died. We grieve and we love. We remember."

Nathalie Himmelrich

I LOST MY PEN

My first trimester flew by. I almost even doubted my status as I had no headache, no morning sickness and no heavy cravings, Due to the wait or excitement of being pregnant or both and many other reasons, I had a fantastic time and just enjoyed being pregnant. During this period, my happiness knew no bounds. One of my husband's friends saw me and told me I was glowing. That pretty much describes how my face was. Mind you, he had no idea I was pregnant but he kept saying there was something different about me.

Five months into my pregnancy (January, 2021), I received the saddest news of all time. My precious biggest cheerleader, the most selfless person ever, my mentor and rock, my dad passed on and the news was broken to me by my husband. I was numb, shocked, broken, devastated, angry and sad. My heart literally broke into a thousand pieces. I mean, how will I go from being the happiest person to the saddest? Anyone that knew my dad knew how jolly, kind, selfless, hardworking (and the list could go on and on) he was. From my birth, this was the lowest point of my life.

On that fateful day my alarm failed to wake me up. I overslept! Generally, I am one of those people that my alarm wakes me up immediately and I never snooze. Alas! That day my alarm didn't wake me up for the first time in my life, I over slept. While asleep, my dad was breathing his last breath.

The only thing that kept me sane was the baby growing in me and my husband's words to me daily. I kept remembering how my dad cried when he heard of my pregnancy and how he told me we were going to have a boy even before we did out gender reveal. My emotions were all over the place. At some point going through this traumatic experience, my obstetrician had to do a couple of tests to ensure I wasn't depressed. I was so angry with God. We waited for seven years and got blessed and four months before I was due, He took my dad. The songs that were on my play list brought back too many painful memories and I had to eventually delete them. Thank God for a supportive and prayerful husband who comforted me and kept sharing God's word with me, for family who stood by me and for friends who understood my mood, gave me space when needed but stayed close with uplifting messages.

In the middle of the pandemic, January 2021, we travelled to Nigeria for my dad's funeral. Looking back now, I was in a daze all through and kept praying for it to be a dream.

Going to Lagos was smooth as it was Covid-19 at its peak so airlines were not flying at full capacity. Everything felt like a dream and it seemed like I was floating. My dad's pillow, wristwatch, some of his shirts and personal belongings seemed like my most prized possessions as I took them back with me so I will always have a part of him. The day I was to return to Canada, the airline official I met at the airport initially didn't want to allow me fly back home because I didn't have a letter from my doctor stating I was fit to return to Canada. My emotions got the better of me and I started yelling at him at the airport. Calming down later, we went to talk to him because he was insisting on us showing a letter from my doctor approving my ability to fly. My tactic changed because being a Saturday and knowing my obstetrician's office in Canada will be closed, I had to tell him my dad passed and the whole story of rushing down to Lagos before he finally let me check in.

Being pregnant and grieving is the most difficult ever. Your hormones are raging and your emotions are all over the place. You just constantly feel like crying. We travelled back to Toronto and time just flew. I was crying so much and was scared at some point. Writing my book became a thing of the past as all the excitement felt before was just gone. The motivation and zeal to continue writing this book left me, I struggled to focus and wished it was a bad dream. I lost my dad and I lost my pen.

Birth

On May 21, 2021, we welcomed our son shine. He weighed 9.9 pounds. Our miracle child. He was born after 7 years of trying to conceive, my husband and I were born in the 7th month of the year, and he was born at 7.21. We named him Oluwabamise (God did it for me), Stephen after his late grandfather. Number 7 till date remains my lucky number.

"There is purpose in your season of waiting."

Megan Smalley

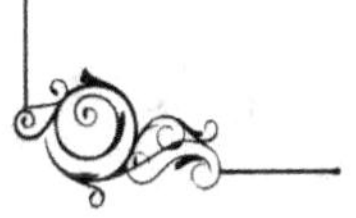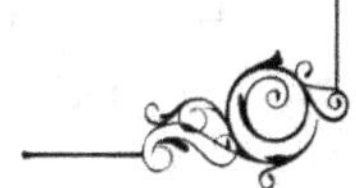

THE 4 SPHERES OF THE JOURNEY

Spiritual:

Spirituality gives a sense of peace and purpose. It is the state of having a connection with God.

I have always believed the Bible is the most important book just as I am sure Muslims believe the Quran is the most important. These books give us the guidelines of our walk with our Maker.

Without faith it is impossible to see God. God is not a person. He exists, but not in our sphere. To believe in him, to hear from him, to even worship him, we need faith and our faith is made stronger by studying the Holy Book.

Our walk with God is spiritual as He is our source, strength, anchor, motivation, peace and hope.

People face seasons of waiting at different times in their lives. It could be for a new job, for breakthrough or in our own case, for a child. In the Bible, Sarah had her baby at 90 years while Rebecca waited for 20 years to give birth to Jacob and Esau. In the process of waiting, one of the most important things is not to give up. It is extremely hard as you may think your prayers can never be answered or what you pray for may look huge.

During my wait, I looked for passages that had to do with waiting and having a child. I read these passages daily and I had such peace that I can't even explain. I knew it wasn't the right time for us to have a baby, I knew God wanted us to have our baby at the right time and in the right place. I started to look up people who waited in the Bible. Stories I knew before, I delved deeper into understanding the story of Hannah (1st Samuel), Sarah (Genesis), Joseph (Genesis 37-50) , Rebecca, Abraham , just to mention a few.

I have always believed that when you pray for something repeatedly for a while, God hears and answers but the 'when' is what we may not be able to comprehend at that time. Think about it, you ask your dad for something, you don't continue disturbing him daily especially when he tells you he has heard, right? After asking God for the same thing, I started to understand the importance of thanksgiving. I knew God had heard and I put on my hat of thanksgiving and started to give Him thanks.

Throughout this journey, certain Bible passages gave me strength. I never knew affirmations were a thing. I had affirmations I said daily.

When we received the good news that I was pregnant, the verse that came to mind was Psalm 126: 1-3

When the Lord turned the captivity of Zion, we were like them that dream. Then was our mouth filled with laughter, and our tongue with singing: then said they among the heathen, The Lord hath done great things for them. The Lord hath done great things for us; whereof we are glad.

2. Physical

The physical aspect of my journey was through exercise. Coincidently, Covid-19 played a part as I worked from home for a few months. I downloaded an app and was exercising religiously without fail.

This period of exercise helped my body. I have always been physically fit but this enhanced my fitness. When exercising, I would play music that resonated with me. My body had to be physically ready to carry this child and I had to be as healthy as possible. I wasn't pregnant when I started exercising but I believed in a healthy lifestyle.

Being a social drinker who occasionally toyed with a glass or 2 at outings, I stopped social drinking.

My husband and I went out a couple of times and it was hilarious when one of our friends thought we were expecting because I refused to drink at a particular outing.

3. Emotional

I found strength in God, my partner who was there with me, my family, my job, friends and engaging in my hobbies.

Protecting yourself emotionally is beneficial to you mentally. Some of the ways to avoid an emotional breakdown is not overdoing pregnancy tests, not allowing your monthly periods get you down, concentrating on self-care, addressing difficult feelings. Talking to someone or writing helps when dealing with infertility. Bear in mind our lives have different aspects. Pregnancy and parenting are one aspect of living. Ensuring a good balance between all these areas help to build a positive and strong mental attitude.

Hence, if we struggle in one aspect or if something is not perfect in one aspect, we have other areas to gain strength from and keep our mentality positive

Although clinic visits can be draining emotionally, especially if you have to go weekly. Going into the clinic gave me hope because entering into the fertility clinic then, we would see so many photos of babies. There was this particular black family's photo, I would always tap into. The photo was right in the middle, the couple reminded me of my husband and I as they were a smiling couple holding their bundle of joy with our fertility doctor. Funny enough, that was one of my highlights visiting the clinic. I would look at all those photos especially the one with the black family and fantasize about holding our own baby and sending our photo to join all those lovely pictures on the wall.

Social

Live your life and don't put a stop to things you would normally do.

It is easy for you to be preoccupied or allow infertility rule your life. We can't always change the circumstances we find ourselves in but we can cope or overcome when faced with challenges.

With us, we continued to live our lives to the extent that some of our friends didn't know we were trying for a baby. They assumed we were still waiting and enjoying life.

Meeting friends, playing games, going out and doing whatever you like doing helps you to live regardless of your pain. I met a lot of women who decided to be in isolation because of the pain of what is not working out yet. This can lead to depression as you spend all that time wishing and thinking while life passes by.

Friends and family are important and they have their roles in our lives. The balance of our social life with work and family gives us positive juice to tap from. Good vibes, good energy and also the flow of information are all advantages of having a good social circle and it's important for our well-being.

"Perseverance is not a long race;
it is many short races one
after the other."

Walter Elliot

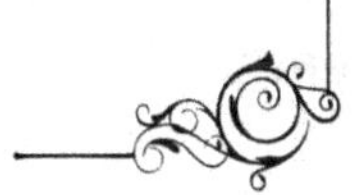

PERSONAL EXPERIENCE OF FIVE WOMEN WHO WENT THROUGH INFERTILITY

Infertility may be God's plan to allow us to journey to achieve His will. It may even be the time to become your husband's best friend. Pardon my perspective, but my personal experience has taught me to always see the positive even in a somewhat negative encounter. Going through infertility can be agonizing and seem unending while being endured.

The stories in this chapter are real life experiences and not fictional. The identities of the women have been replaced with pseudonyms for privacy. The purpose is to share and highlight different journeys as there are multiple ways people are affected by infertility.

These women are strong, beautiful and blessed as they went through the difficult period of infertility but came out victorious. It details their struggle with fertility and how they balanced it with family, friends, societal pressure etc. These are stories that will give you goose bumps and make you shed a tear while also steering up your faith.

Kim's story

We got married in September 2011. We weren't bothered about fertility or infertility because everything seemed fine, I had regular periods, felt healthy, we had sex regularly, and all was well. After two years of marriage and there was no pregnancy, we decided to see a doctor. We were referred to a gynaecologist who advised us to take some tests. He said he'd carry out HSG on me. *HSG is an X-ray test to outline the internal shape of the uterus and show whether the fallopian tubes are blocked. In HSG, a thin tube is threaded through the vagina and cervix. A substance known as contrast material is injected into the uterus.*

However, this procedure is extremely painful. What was inserted into my vagina wasn't thin and wasn't lubricated. I screamed the whole hospital down and personally thought I was going to pass out. He also carried out tests on my husband's sperm. Checked the motility rate and the sperm count, then he said hubby had low motility rate and my fallopian tubes were blocked. He said and I quote "you can never get pregnant, there's really nothing you can do, even if you try IVF". Didn't that seem like it was all over? I cried and my husband was sad. It got to us and we were cold to each other for about two days and then we bounced back.

Continued like we never heard what that horrible doctor told us.

Fast forward to a few months after, we visited another doctor who was upset with the first doctor for not carrying out other tests before HSG. He mentioned we'd be taking different tests for both me and my husband. *He suggested Folliculometry. It is an ultrasound examination during which the number and size of follicles is determined. It is performed repeatedly, because of the growth of follicles and prediction or evidence of ovulation. A follicle grows about 1-2 mm per day and ovulation starts once it reaches 18-30 mm.* This test we never did, but he had a lot of medication for us. He had asked questions and requested for results done in the past. The doctor placed us on weekly medication, when we got tired, we stopped without discussing it.

After that we got information of a medical doctor that had diversified into trado-medicine or should we call it Naturopathic medicine. She was interviewed on the radio and my friend sent the number to me. Well, we called her and went over to see her. She had requested we visit with all scan results, tests results and whatever it is we had. We headed over there and she said she'd work with the doctor that had said I had blocked fallopian tubes. However, our first treatment was cleansing of the body system. She gave some herbs and we took them. I think it really did some detoxification because we felt lighter but we never went back for the next treatment. It didn't sit right with us so we let it go and just relaxed.

Years passed and we still took life easy. I had people say to me to come to certain churches and once I mentioned I was going to tell my husband, they advised against that. They'd ask what I'd do if my husband refused to come and refused me going, I said I'd listen to him because we were in it together; they all concluded I wasn't ready to have a child.

Then my husband's aunty referred us to a gynecologist. This was the doctor she had used for years. She had given birth to all her children there. Her first child at that time was in her late twenties so we knew the doctor had to have a lot of experience.

We headed there with all documents and said we would be seeing the MD and no one else. We saw him; he checked everything and confirmed that he knew the doctor we had seen (the first doctor that carried out the HSG). He asked if we agree with the doctor, we said NO. We insisted on starting afresh as we didn't want any recycling. He confirmed he'd still carry out the HSG however, his process was different and could be expensive. We agreed to go ahead.

His own process was going to knock me off so I don't feel the pain and that way he could get a more accurate result. While conducting HSG, the patient is expected not to move (how do you stay still while in pain?) So we went ahead and got the HSG done, well, guess what. My tubes were not blocked.

He did the Folliculometry for me and tests on my hubby, everything came back fine. He said all we needed was to wait and that it was obviously not yet time. He advised we keep having sex and calm down. That was in 2016; by 2017 December I was pregnant. We had our first child in September 2018 (on our 7th wedding anniversary), and had the second child in January 2021.

We really just needed to wait. I mean check out how I got pregnant with the second one. Just constant headaches and missed periods and I was confirmed pregnant. Everything works at the right time.

I had people send me messages that I was "doing fine girl" instead of me to go and get pregnant. Another friend told me she could help us with pregnancy, thinking it was surrogacy she wanted to offer, alas, she wanted to sleep with my hubby. A male friend offered his services to me too, claiming I look very fertile so it shouldn't be an issue. People would heap responsibilities on me at work stating that they couldn't give the junior staff that got married years after me because that junior staff had children and I didn't. Friends told me they couldn't start 'ajo'- thrift collection with me because they had responsibilities and I didn't because I had no child. WRONG, so WRONG.

So many comments while trying to conceive and even after conceiving, I still had painful comments. Some people never saw me pregnant so they whispered it must have been another child…we overcame and we're still standing.

The above questions and comments shouldn't be dished out to women trying to conceive, it's already hard on them, why make it harder?

It was okay to wish me a happy mother's day while trying for a baby, but that's me, it may not be okay with the next lady. It was okay to pray for me and pray with me. It wasn't okay to keep asking me 'how far'.

For me, IVF and adoption should come from the couple and not outside the couple. All these stages and processes could be very emotional and how each woman handles it is the right way for her.

Every trip to the hospital during this time should be made by both the man and woman. Nothing like it's the woman that would carry the pregnancy and so she needs it more. They should both visit the specialist together.

Above all, the woman's health and frame of mind is very important. Having a supportive husband and supportive in-laws is perfect for a woman trying to conceive. Not for one day did my in-laws ask me 'how far'. They prayed for me and never looked down on me. They visited often; some lived with us and still do. They were with us and never said I wasn't a woman for not having a child. I'm super thankful.

Sylvia's Story

I got married in 2014. When we got married we decided to wait a bit before having babies. In my opinion waiting for 2 to 3 years in order to build my banking career was a good choice and my husband agreed.

After three years we were finally ready to start making babies however it wasn't forthcoming so we started seeking medical interventions. I did series of test and procedures ranging from HSG to Tubular flushing to hormonal profile MIR and a whole lot more.

All these procedures came back positive except the hormonal profile. It showed I had hormonal imbalance meaning my prolactin levels were really high and this made me lactate like a breast feeding mum. With this, it was hard to conceive because my body was responding to the fact that I had a baby and made it difficult to conceive. From there we started going from one hospital to the other looking for a lasting solution. The first gynecologist we met treated us. After months of no results we moved to another then to another.

As at September 2018 which made it of our 4th year of marriage I had met with 4 top gynecologists in Lagos and yet no results.

My mother In-law was worried and put a call through to us for a meeting. Apparently she spoke to a friend of hers who mentioned to her that we should try IVF (In vitro fertilization) we were open to the suggestion and decided to give it a try.

We started IVF procedure the same month. The 30 day cycle of injection, egg extraction and transfer of eggs back. At the end of the cycle, 3 embryos were transferred back to my ovaries and a week later I was confirmed pregnant with twins. That felt like the best moment of our lives.

Finally it had happened "hallelujah". We were super excited about this news and was willing to share this good news with anyone who wanted to listen.

The pregnancy progressed and during the first trimester I coped with the morning sickness and constant headaches. After the first trimester I started my antenatal and that felt like the best moment of our lives. God had indeed giving us double for the trouble right. That's how we felt.

At 20 weeks I was advised by my gynecologist at the same hospital I did the IVF to perform a cervical cerclage procedure since I was having twins. We gladly agreed as we wanted to do everything possible to protect our precious twins. At 21 weeks the cerclage procedure was done. After the procedure I was fine for a few days then started bleeding. Being in my second trimester I wasn't supposed to be bleeding not even with the cerclage done however the bleeding was heavy and I was rushed back to the hospital.

After spending a week at the hospital, it was discovered that the twins had shared one placenta making them identical twins and the placenta was not attached to my womb a condition called "placenta previa". I was advised to be on bed rest for the remaining five months of pregnancy and was told the birth would be through CS. This posed a major risk to the pregnancy and my survival. We started praying about it and hoping for the best.

One evening while on admission at the hospital I started bleeding heavily again, the doctor came and told me he had no choice than to loosen the cerclage and induce me for labour. Before responding, the doctor induced me and I was in labour, I gave birth to the twins (a boy and a girl) with tears in my eyes and pain in my heart. They were so tiny and lifeless and it felt like all hope was lost again.

My husband rushed down to the hospital that night at 2 am and he just had to be strong for me. I cried and cried and later told myself it's time to move on.

After a month I finally went back to work. Some of my colleagues at work accused me of not inviting them to the naming ceremony while some who knew what happened kept looking at me with pity. There was little I could say as I was grieving but needed to get my life back. Time they say heals and am thankful that with time I was able to move on and kept praying to God because He knows best.

A year passed by and nothing happened. No pregnancy as we wished. Having heard and read stories of those who got pregnant after their IVF procedure, our prayer was for a miracle but it didn't happen.

Two years after the incident I got a call from a doctor in Lagos who said he got my number from a friend and wanted to see me.

Prior to this time I had blocked myself from having any fertility conversation with my friends and family. This was our sixth year of marriage and we would put up a defense when anyone concerned tried to speak to us about conception as we believed we had our own fair share already.

Back to the doctor who called me, apparently a junior colleague of mine who was concerned shared my story with him and he felt he should reach out. She begged the doctor not to mention her name as she was so sure I won't take it easy with her. This doctor kept calling me every month and I will decline his calls and ignore his messages.

Finally, year 2020 came and it was a lock down year. I and my husband had decided that we will just go with the flow and not bow to any pressure from our parents. Prior to the lock down my husband's god-mother had summoned us for a meeting at her house and she suggested to us that we should go for "adoption" since the pregnancy wasn't forth coming. In her words "Ori omo lo ma pe omo wa aye" meaning having a child around you might be a roadmap to my conception. I cried my eyes out on that day as I remembered the twins we lost.

My husband and I agreed it hadn't gotten to that yet. Maybe if we try for ten years then we can start thinking of adopting a child.

After that day I told my husband about the gynecologist who had been calling and sending me messages and asked my husband to let us give him a try after the lock down. That will be our 6th gynecologist by the way and my husband agreed.

When the lockdown was eased, we went to see the gynecologist in Ebute Metta in Lagos. He told us to go back and run some tests which we had done before. I reluctantly agreed. One of those test was HSG which on the second procedure revealed that my left tube was blocked and just the right one is free.

Oh my world came crashing down. The sad part is that the high prolactin was still present. I kept asking how one tube will be blocked, my tubes were okay before now what could have happened and so much more on my mind.

I think God was just telling me according to His word in 1 Corinthians 1 vs 27 KJV
"But God hath chosen the foolish things of the world to confound the wise; and God hath chosen the weak things of the world to confound the things which are mighty;"

Indeed everything will work out in God's time. The doctor told me to put my trust in God and suggested he placed me on medications for three months and if nothing happens we can think of a procedure we could do. Even my husband was in doubt as he told the doctor that he is not sure I could conceive naturally looking at my medical history and the fact that one tube is blocked. The doctor told us one free tube is even more than enough and we should put our trust in God. He placed me on some medication which I had used some years back and I kept on arguing with him that I don't think this will work and he should give me something stronger.

The gynecologist encouraged me to use the medication for 3 cycles and if they don't work he will give me something stronger. I agreed and started the medications with prayers. This was September 2021. By the third month I realized I had missed my period for November and took a home pregnancy test on the

31st day. Behold I got double lines I was pregnant for the first time in my life and It happened naturally isn't God wonderful. So this could happen to me even with my one tube left.

His word says in Habakkuk 2:3 "for the vision is yet for an appointed time, but at the end it shall speak, and not lie though it tarry wait for it; because it shall surely come, it will not tarry'.

God makes all things beautiful at his time. My pregnancy was so smooth, no morning sickness nor swollen foot no pre-eclampsia nor "placenta previa". I had the best and smoothest 9 months journey. The sweetest part was one could hardly tell I was pregnant in my first and second trimester. I also got my US visa application approved even at 6 month pregnant against all odds.

On the 11th of August 2021, I welcomed my baby boy at Oak Bend Medical Center, Houston, Texas. He is so strong and healthy weighing 3.78kg at birth. I named him OLUWAJOMILOJU meaning "God Surprised me" he is indeed God's gift to us as he made our lives so beautiful. He is the cutest baby ever, came with a lot of hair and the cutest little smile. Indeed what God cannot do does not exist. We humans can only try, God will perfect all at his appointed time.

Are you reading my story and still waiting, keep trusting God He will come through for you too for his word says none shall be barren. Genesis 1 vs 28 Be fruitful and multiple and replenish the earth and subdue it. He will definitely come through for you. Amen.

Lyan's Story

My fertility story is more than a story but a testimony that I am always willing to share to inspire others. I started trying for a baby in 2013 after getting married in 2012. I eventually got pregnant in 2016 (4years) my very first pregnancy ever, it was just a miracle. The journey started when I relocated to the UK to join my husband, I received a letter from my local hospital that I needed to attend the chest clinic because the X-ray that was done at the airport showed that my chest was not clear. During assessment the nurse asked if I was pregnant that

my abdomen is bulky and feels hard to touch, a referral was done to do an ultrasound of the abdomen that revealed I had multiple fibroids. I had myomectomy done in 2014. Fifteen (15) fibroids were taken out. We waited for about a year and there was still no sign of pregnancy. IVF was advised by my doctor. Referral was made to another hospital and my first appointment was in December 2015 with a scan showing new fibroids growing which means I could have another surgery before starting treatment. This made me break down and I remember crying all the way home, but my husband kept on saying have you lost your faith? The doctor told me to go and enjoy my Christmas and call the clinic after my menstrual period in January to enable them carry out a more invasive procedure. In January, I waited and waited, my period was not forthcoming. For the first time in my life I did a pregnancy test, and it was positive. It was unbelievable, I kept on repeating the test to be sure I was pregnant. When I told my husband it was the happiest moment of our lives.

No societal pressure at all, not a lot of family interference other than family friends that have been in the same position advising on steps to take. Physically I was good, going for medical appointments was a time of reflection for me. However, as a couple we tried to enjoy every moment but to be honest at some point during the journey, it felt like there was no point having sex. I was emotionally unstable and always in my corner because I did not want anyone to ask or even advise me on the subject matter. But generally, I would say everyone was supportive to the best of their ability.

Ife's Story

I waited for six years before I had my rainbow baby after four miscarriages. Looking back, going to a boarding school in Nigeria, my period was almost nonexistent. I started my period at the age of 9 and it was never consistent. Being diagnosed with PCOS at an early age of 18. My doctor prescribed pills for me which I continued to use until I got married.

I got married at 23 and stopped taking the pills hoping my period would return or I'd get pregnant but nothing happened. At 24 I was diagnosed with Hypothyroidism. Four years later, we went to a fertility clinic and was told I was not ovulating. After a series of treatments simulating my ovulation with Letrozole, within 1 year of the treatment I got pregnant three times. The pregnancies were lost at 6 weeks, 10 weeks and 19 weeks. Those were the worst days of my life. As a couple, we were determined to make it work and keep trying. During the pandemic we paid for an IUI. I got pregnant immediately and I had a beautiful baby girl. This journey is difficult and only my faith in God and love from my spouse and family got me through. The doctors were knowledgeable and helped me every step of the way.

Rebecca's Story

When we got married, we planned not to have any kids yet for the first two years, as we were not physically and mentally ready, so we decided to go on birth control.

About two years into the marriage, we were finally ready for kids and started trying to conceive, but no luck.

We sought medical advice and were told that one of the side effects of birth control pills is that in some cases, it takes about a year for the effects to wear off, which meant I had about a year to wait before I could conceive.

Even though the information was upsetting, it gave me some form of comfort that nothing was wrong and the delay was as a result of the birth control.

Another year passed and nothing had changed. The effect of the birth control must have worn off, so what could be causing the delay this time? We started to get worried and anxious.

When nothing happened, we decided to seek medical advice.

We had to undergo a series of fertility tests, most of which were unpleasant. The results came out fine and I was told we had no fertility issues, so what could be causing the delay? This made me even more anxious and upset.

We kept trying, praying and believing that God's time is the best and it would happen someday.
One thing I ensured is that the circumstance did not affect my mood as I kept a level head always.

Of course, there was a lot of concerns from the parents and they would often consult several doctors on our behalf.

In the process of waiting, we had to develop thick skin as different people would often give advice and everyone had something to say, also considering the part of the world we live in where it's the norm for women to conceive as soon as they get married.

Also at work, colleagues would give me advice, some of which was to try IVF, but I would usually just say "okay" to them, and not allow their advice and opinions get to me.

The waiting period was emotionally draining for me as every month, I would hope and pray I'll miss a period, but it was always disappointing.

Six years into our marriage, I finally conceived, after about 4 years of trying and waiting.

It felt unbelievable when I went to the hospital for a pregnancy test and the result came out positive. I remember how I couldn't contain my joy and quickly called my parents to inform them.

In 2016, we welcomed our bundle of joy, and it just felt like the perfect timing. I believe God has his reason for everything, the delays and the experience of waiting, and now believe that a delay does not necessarily mean a denial.

"He made a Way."

Travis Greene

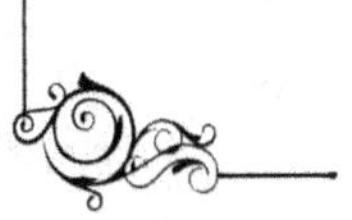 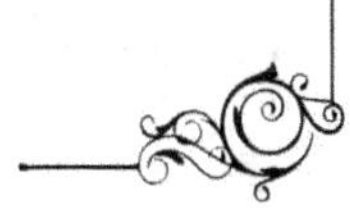

INFERTILITY- A TWO WAY STREET- A HIS AND HERS JOURNEY

There is a stereotype with infertility as it pertains more towards women. The journey of infertility even if it's one party that is infertile is burdened by both partners. The man is not exempt. Most men have developed a tough skin as the pressure is mainly towards the woman. My husband did face his own fair share. We went through the burden together but we experienced it differently. Here is the journey from his perspective.

The male narrative or perspective doesn't seem to be a best seller in fertility stories. When many hear fertility, it essentially points at the woman and conception but frankly it affects men too. This version of the story is not about male infertility but rather my experience as a husband going through that journey of fertility with my wife of seven years.

We got married in December of 2014 and never for once thought we would not have kids soon after. To be fair, we lived in different countries and met occasionally. She was a teacher in Dubai and I had a regional sales role in West Africa. One advantage of our jobs that helped the long- distance was the privilege of travel. As a teacher, she had lots of holidays which meant she would take long trips for the long and short holidays while i also did the same whenever I had to travel. We were at this stage for about 2 years. It was all fun and bliss as we loved our time together and looked forward to a nearby future where we would not live apart.

Fast forward to about two years after, I quit my job as I was not eligible for a transfer due to my tenure and I relocated to Dubai to be with my wife, start an MBA programme and hopefully start a family. At this period, there was no pressure or any thoughts of something being wrong, we just thought we didn't do it enough (have enough sex).

So the hard work began, 'you never know how much work sex can be until you are trying for a baby'. At this point I was being advised to time her ovulation period and seriously hammer my wife. I didn't need to time anything I was always ready, we were at it constantly, sometimes it took the fun out of it because it felt like a chore.

After a while, our concerns rose but still no pressure. We decided to seek help and that's how the visits started. The first specialist saw me separately and ran a series of test. This was after my wife had done a fibroid surgery. She still did not conceive and they thought I should get checked as well. The doctor prescribed some medication after test results showed low sperm counts/slow motility of swimmers. I felt bad as I always thought I was fine but felt better realising the problem was about to solved. I started taking the drugs, some effervescent powder I would mix with water or a drink and consume twice daily. I started getting impatient after a while as the Doctor did not tell how long I was to continue and these drugs were not particularly cheap so I stopped taking them while she continued a series of treatments.

On the flip side my prayer life was inconsistent as I went through a unique phase. Emotionally, we seemed okay about the whole fertility drama maybe because our families were total blessings to us.

Without me saying much, my parents never made my wife uncomfortable. I remember it was my dad who would ask me about the progress. He would say in my native tongue, 'se o ti wole'? Meaning, has it entered? Lol. I remember a day I brought up the topic with my mom, and she immediately sat upright eagerly to hear me out and offer her support. She was shocked as I had never talked about it with her like that generally and this was me bringing it up by myself. She was supportive and offered prayers and was glad we had decided to talk to a specialist and not just wait it out.

My dad was the one who would regularly ask if she was pregnant and at the end of the Q&A, he would prophesy and say a prayer.

Emotionally, we seemed to handle ourselves well and we would talk about how we felt and even fantasize about kids. I would occasionally joke about wanting 7 kids, and everyone would laugh at me saying, wait till you have your first I bet you will rescind that thought. One weird part was the assumption from many friends and associate who thought we were not ready for kids. Maybe due to the fact that many people went through depression or were lethargic in their dealings, or simply disinterested in general affairs or even withdrawn. I commend my wife who after all these drama and surgery decided to join the children's' church to enable her teach and even draw nearer to kids even though her day job already involved children. Frankly, it was tough considering the period it took us to eventually have one. Looking back now, those days are forgotten, I hardly remember how I felt but I know I am grateful. Grateful to the friends who were sensitive to the pain, grateful to family for being dependable and comforting, grateful to my wife for being strong and holding up the faith and grateful to God for keeping his promises.

This journey has been long as the baby came in the 7th year of marriage. I hardly remember some details but I know it was a tough and lonely journey. Prayers went up, answers came down eventually. I cannot remember how many alter calls for miracles we responded to or how many times pastors laid their hands on our heads and on my wife's belly. I believe in prayers and I believe God responded but the miracle was for an appointed time.

My testimony: In August 2020, my dear sister called and encouraged me as I had confided in her about my prayer life and how I was inconsistent. She mentioned a prayer platform she joined and how she was able to pray better. I agreed to join for the purpose of having a better prayer life and miraculously, the month after, we were pregnant. What God cannot do does not exist. The shock of conception was quite overwhelming and I can still remember the moment we got a call from the doctor's office and how speechless we were when we got off the phone. The miracle had happened. We had waited for about 7 years and it happened just like that. We looked at each other and we could not even cry. We just smiled and felt our faith get stronger

This is my testimony, our road to fertility, our tears and pain regarding one aspect of our lives, our journey through it all and our thanksgiving as we endured and yet overcame and achieved that which almost seemed impossible. It happened for us in Gods time, it will happen for you as well.

Tip- Men, the journey is spiritual and emotional, we must be the rock for our wives

-We must seek help and talk to the right people

-We must develop a tough skin, people will say insensitive things and we cannot react to everything

-we must not be too sensitive, not everyone means bad as the words may not come as intended.

-We serve a living God and He moves in mysterious ways.

GLOSSARY

This chapter mainly contains the definitions of medical terms given when going infertility. You get accustomed to acronyms and definitions of words using to describe various stages.

Fertility

According to American pregnancy association, Fertility is the natural capability to conceive.

Infertility

According to Canada.ca, Although there is no single definition of the term infertility, it typically refers to a lack of conception after a reasonable period of sexual intercourse without contraception (one year for women who are under 35 years, 6 months for women over 35 years).

The second type of infertility is called 'Secondary infertility'.

Secondary infertility on the other hand is when you have trouble conceiving or carrying a pregnancy to term after successfully getting pregnant at least once before.

Primary and secondary infertility usually share the same causes.

Infertility can affect both men and women.

What is TTC?
Trying to Conceive in relation to fertility forums is more about the research, patience and entire journey involved in preparing to become pregnant.

Ultrasound

Ultrasound is a procedure that uses high-frequency sound waves to view internal structures of the body. Ultrasound is used during pregnancy to check that your baby is healthy. Gotten from itttfertilitycentre. org.uk

IUI

This is known as intrauterine insemination (IUI) It is a type of artificial insemination. Sperm that have been washed/prepared and concentrated are placed directly in your uterus around the time your ovary releases one or more eggs to be fertilized.it is inserted through a soft catheter (Source: mayoclinic.org).

IVF

IVF is a medical procedure whereby an egg is fertilized by sperm in a test tube or elsewhere outside the body.

Fibroids

Fibroids are common benign tumours of smooth muscle in the uterus (womb)

HSG

According to medicinenet.com, a hysterosalpingogram is a procedure that uses an x-ray to examine the cavity of the uterus and fallopian tubes. It is performed for the diagnosis of infertility.

Sonohsterogram

It is a procedure to look at the inside of the uterus.

Cervical Cerclage

It is a procedure that helps keep a pregnant woman's cervix from opening too soon before delivery.

PCOS

Polycystic ovary syndrome (PCOS) is a condition in which the ovaries produce an abnormal amount of androgens, male sex hormones that are usually present in women in small amounts.